Table of Contents

Romantic Scents

Welcome to the book on romantic scents. This wonderful world of *aromantics* will have your lover hot on your heels for love and passion. Wear one of the perfumes out on a special date. Or use the oils around the home for that special night. Why not? You have been to the right restaurant, bought the right meal, picked up the house and laid your beds with clean sheets. But what about scent. Don't forget to add that little extra touch with some of the *aromantics* in this book. With Twenty luscious blends you're bound to find something you love in this book. Whether it be a new perfume of your own branding, or simply to make the living room give off a welcoming smell when you enter. Oils can be smelt via an oil burner or diffuser, filled with some of the beautiful essential oils used in this book. You will find the blends within both please and excite you and your partner.

Essential oils are extracted from plants using steam or hydro distillation.

Absolutes are typically used in perfumery rather than for aromatherapy. They are extracted using chemical solvents and step two, with ethyl alcohol.

Essential oils should be stored in dark cool places in **amber** or **cobalt** blue coloured bottles, to prevent them from going off or evaporating[1].

The oils have notes, just like in music. some oils are top notes, some are middle and some are base. These are outlined in a table at the end of this book under the oils and their properties for use in this book.

---

[1]http://www.edenbotanicals.com/essential-oils-pure-therapeutic-grade.html (Accessed 1/07/11)

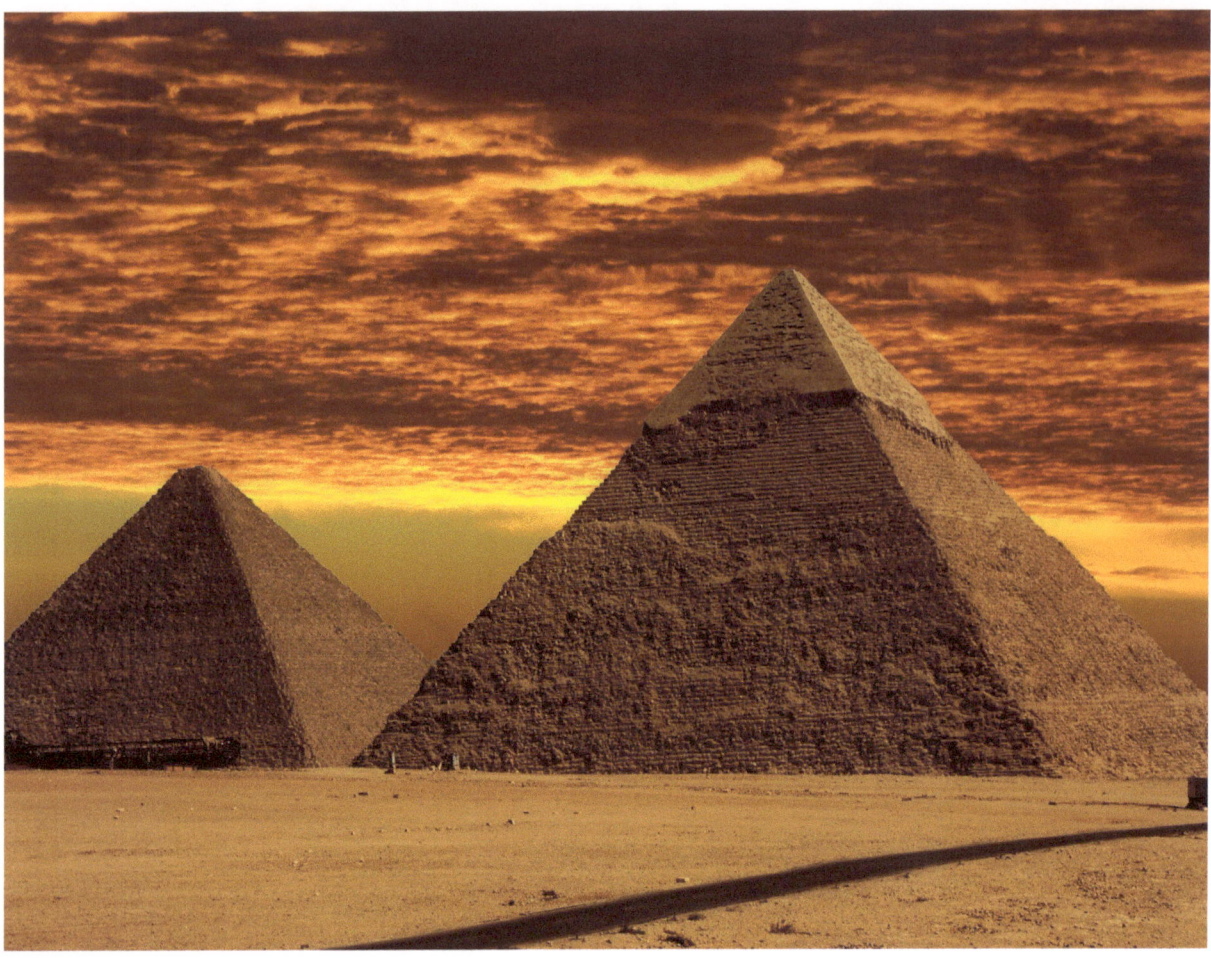

Photo: Pyramids of Egypt, Windowseat, photoxpress.com

<u>History of Aromatherapy</u>

Aromatherapy, (noun), is *The use of aromatic oils obtained from plants for healing or to promote well being*[2].

Since ancient times, lovers have been using scent to increase their attractiveness and woo their beloved. *Aromantics* are scents derived form aroma-therapeutic essential oils, which woo, entice and excite lovers. Aromatherapy is rooted in the Greek words for fragrance and treatment. It was named by the French chemist René Maurice Gattefossé in the 1920's, who discovered that lavender had pain relief and healing properties. The ancient Egyptians used scent to attract and heal. During celebrations and rituals, they wore cones of scented substance on their heads that would melt in the sun and release beautiful aromas. Men and woman wore scents just as they do today. They also used fragrant oils for embalming the dead such as

---

[2]Waitem M., ed, 2007,Oxford Dictionary and Thesaurus, Oxford, Oxford University Press.

cedarwood, clove, cinnamon, nutmeg and myrrh. The scent could still be detected when the mummies were opened and examined in the twentieth century[3].

Cleopatra scented her boat sails with Jasmine. Jasmine, today is considered to be one of the foremost oils for sensuality. She had priest perfumers who exclusively invented perfumes for her. Interesting to note that the Latin word for perfume is 'perfumer' which means 'through smoke'. Even today we burn our essential oils in an oil burner. When Cleopatra wrapped herself in a carpet and unrolled herself from it to surprise Caesar she was steeped in heady aromatic scents[4] and Caesar fell for her.

From Egypt the art of aromatherapy spread to Greece and later Europe. Although it saw a decline in the middle ages when disease was regarded by the church as being a punishment from God. Greek doctors travelled to Egypt and brought back knowledge of aromatherapy with them. Greece had a medical school on the island of Cos, where Hippocrates taught. He said "The way to health is to have an aromatic bath and a scented massage every day."[5] Later in Rome they used aroma's for a number of purposes, including bath-houses, massage and around the home.

Of course in China they have been using incense since ancient times. Aromatherapy probably began in China at the same time as in Ancient Egypt. An ancient Chinese medical book dated from 2700 BC listed over 300 aromatic herbs[6]. Similarly in India, in ancient times they used sandalwood and incense for religious and celebratory purposes.

By the 17th C. More than 60 essential oils were known and being used. During the terrible black plague during the middle ages, perfumers were spared from it, due to their close proximity to the oils. Residents of Bucklersbury in England and other certain geographical areas, were also spared from the plague because of the fields of lavender that grew there[7].

Aromatherapy has enjoyed a more scientific method of analyses during the 20th century. It is still very popular in Europe. In the United states it is mainly used for recreational purposes. In South America in Ecuador essential oils are researched in hospitals. Aromatherapy has it's cynics. In most of the West it is considered to be a complimentary modality only and not as a replacement for modern drugs. Yet some take it very seriously and research continues into this unique therapy with more interesting developments to come, for eg. The distillation of new plant species from the Amazon rainforest for the purpose of aromatherapy and medicine.

---

[3]http://www.aromatherapypoint.com/history-of-aromatherapy/ (Accessed 1/6/11)
[4]http://theida.com/aromatic-plants/love-potion-by-kris-wrede (Accessed 1/6/11)
[5]http://www.essential-oils-lifestyles.com/aromatherapy-history.html (Accessed 1/06/11)
[6]http://www.essentials-of-aromatherapy.com/history_of_aromatherapy.html (Accessed 1/06/11)
[7]http://www.essential-oils-lifestyles.com/aromatherapy-history-2.html (Accessed 2/06/11)

How Aromatherapy Works

Aromatherapy is simply the use of essential plant oils to improve mental and physical well being. Although there are a lot of cynics, aromatherapy has been well researched and is often accepted widely, even in some hospitals. Aromatherapy is said to be an emotional, sensuous sensation that bypasses the left, logical side of the brain to the more emotional right side, via your sense of smell. The aromas reach the olfactory bulb in the brain and spread to certain neurons, causing a chemical reaction. For example Lavender increases the happiness chemical, serotonin and causes a tranquillising affect. Lavender is great for stress and general well being[8].

Essential oils can also enter via skin follicles and entering the blood stream during topical application such as during a massage. Beware of contraindications (IE: when you should not use topical oils) such as broken skin or any rash. You also shouldn't use it during the first trimester of pregnancy and you should use a weaker concentration of the oils in the other trimesters.

---

[8] http://www.youtube.com/watch?v=kNHVAWnXr1E (Accessed 5/06/11)

Aromatherapy Contraindications

1. Never take essential oils internally.
2. Never apply the essential oils neat to the skin.
3. Do not use whilst pregnant
4. Do not use on children (especially those under 5).
5. Always dilute the oils really well before use.
6. Keep away from eyes and mucous membranes
7. For the purposes outlined in this book do not use in doses over 10 ml.
8. Extreme care should be taken if the patient is receiving chemotherapy, it could trigger nausea.
9. Before using a specific oil a simple patch test should be done to ensure freedom from allergies. (any effect will be immediate).
10. Check with your doctor about using aromatherapy if you are on other medications, usually it is safe.
11. Beware of sunlight after using on skin. Some oils especially citrus oils can cause photo-sensitivity.

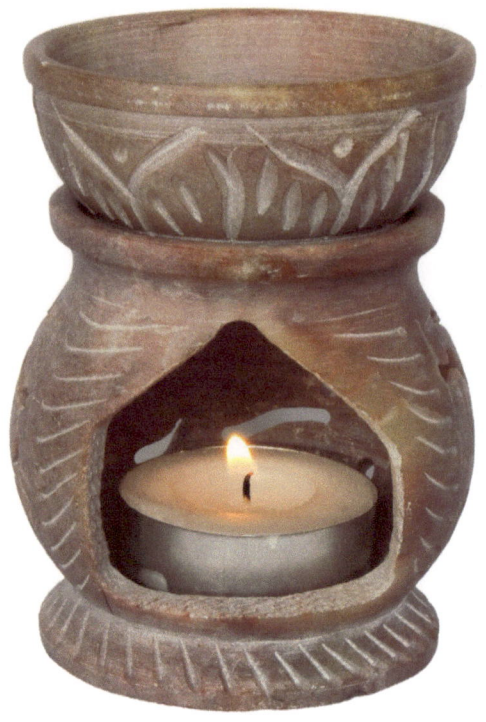

Photo: Oil burner, loznnisS, photoxpress.com

How to Use the Oils.

1. Oil burner (do not leave this burning unattended)
2. Massage Oil
3. Perfume
4. Scented handkerchief
5. Potpourri
6. Spray bottle with water base
7. In the washing machine
8. Add to soaps
9. Add to candles
10. In the bath
11. In a steam bowl (be careful this can be quite strong)
12. Bath Bombs
13. Bath Crystals
14. Scented cotton ball

Recipe Blends

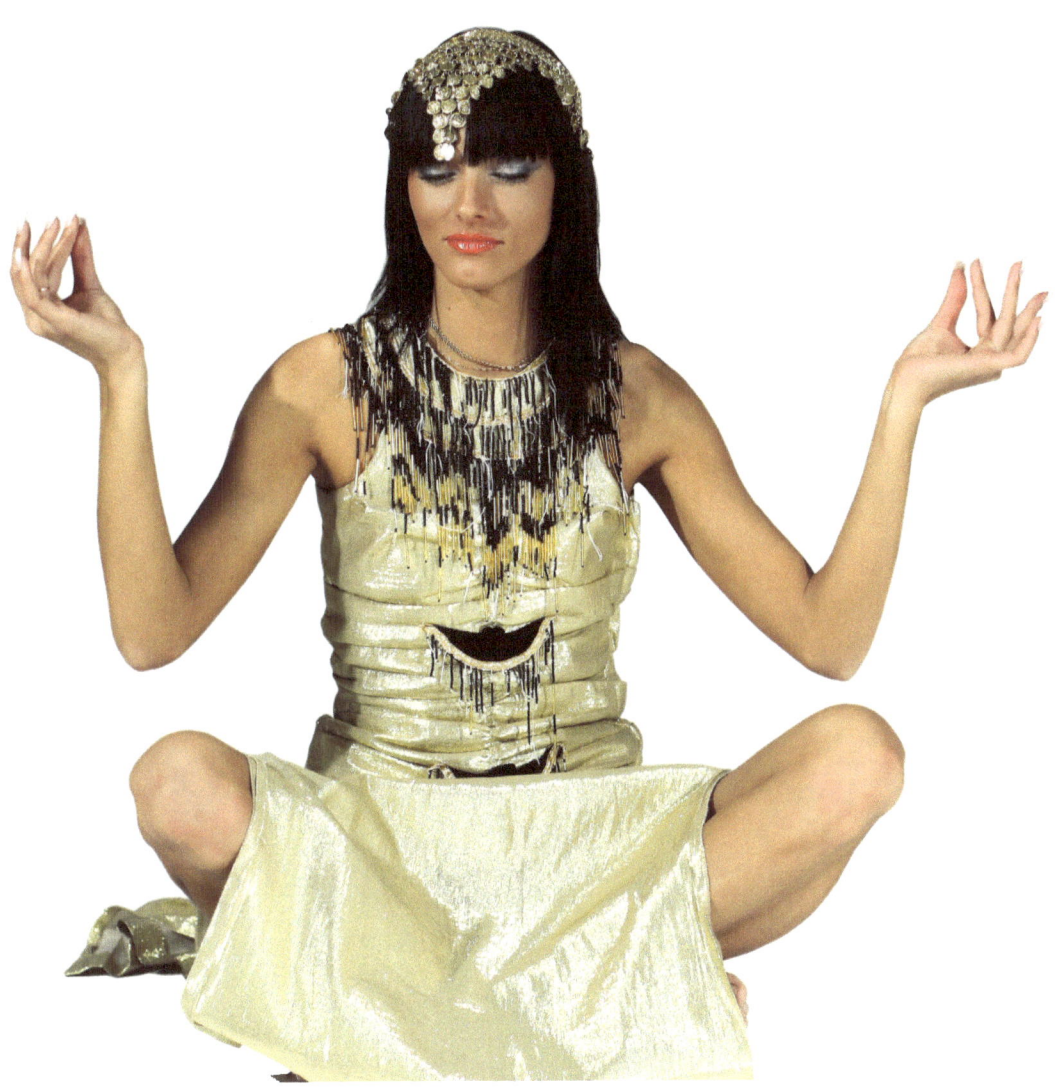

Photo: Cleopatra model, Dreef, photoxpress.com

Cleopatra eau de parfum[9]

50 drops Blood Orange
25 drops Lemon
18 drops Jasmine Sambac
 7 drops Ylang Ylang
13 drops Rose Absolute
5 drops Blue Lotus
11 drops Myrtle
8 drops Cinnamon
12 drops Vanilla

Place in a 30ml (one ounce) bottle in a base perfumer's alcohol, (You can use Vodka, just don't drink it!) or in an unscented Jojoba base, to be used as a perfume oil.

Oriental 'O'

(for oil burner)

5 drops Rose
4 drops Jasmine
3 drops mandarin[10]

Place in a base of some water in an oil burner.

Eastern Flare

(For oil burner)

3 drops rose,
3 drops sandalwood,
2 drops mandarin[11]

Place in a base of some water in an oil burner.

---

[9]http://theida.com/aromatic-plants/love-potion-by-kris-wrede (accessed 1/6/11)
[10]http://www.zimbio.com/Aromatherapy/articles/56/Aphrodisiac+aromas+top+scents+temptation (accessed 3/06/11)
[11]http://www.zimbio.com/Aromatherapy/articles/56/Aphrodisiac+aromas+top+scents+temptation (accessed 3/06/11)

Femme Fatal

2 drops Clary Sage,
4 drops Jasmine
2 drops Neroli
4 drops Rose Otto
3 drops Rosewood
4 drops Sandalwood
2 drops Tangerine
4 Ylang Ylang

Place the oils in an oil burner, bath or massage oil base such as Jojoba or Almond. This one is really raunchy, so, be prepared.

Male Rapture

4 drops cedarwood
2 drops Clary Sage
4 drops Frankincense
4 drops Jasmine
4 drops Rosewood
4 drops Sandalwood
4 drops Vetiver
4 drops Ylang Ylang.

Place in oil burner, bath or massage oil base such as Jojoba or Almond.

Three Aromantics[12]

One

2 drops Clary Sage
2 drops Neroli
4 drops Patchouli

Two

4 drops Patchouli
4 drops Sandalwood
4 drops Ylang Ylang

---

[12]http://www.suite101.com/content/great-sex--boost-sexual-desire-and-intensity-with-aromatherapy-a279844 (Accessed 3/6/11)

Three

2 drops Clary Sage
4 drops Rose
4 drops Sandalwood

Place the oils in an oil burner, bath or massage oil base such as Jojoba or Almond.

Romance Body Wash[13].

Ingredient List:
- 1 part concentrated Castille soap
- 1 part water
- 1 tablespoon of almond oil
- 20-30 drops of your favorite essential oil(s).

\
Combine in an 250ml/ 8oz bottle

Step 1: Add the almond oil.
Step 2: Add the essential oils and gently swirl to mix.
Step 3: Add the water – this is as simple as filling the bottle half full of water.
Step 4: Add the castille soap until the bottle is almost full.

Once you have combined all of the ingredients, gently shake the bottle to mix.

Pleasure Parfum

2 drops Bergamot
2 drops Grapefruit
4 drops Jasmine
2 drops Woody violet
4 drops Sandalwood.

Place the oils in a base oil of Jojoba or Almond and used sparingly in your favourite way.

---

[13]http://www.mommahealth.com/a-chemical-free-healthy-baby-body-wash-to-clean-your-skin.htm

Too Hot to Handle

2 drops Clary Sage
4 drops Sandalwood
4 drops Ylang Ylang

Place the oils in a base oil of Johoba or Almond and used sparingly in your favourite aromatherapy method.

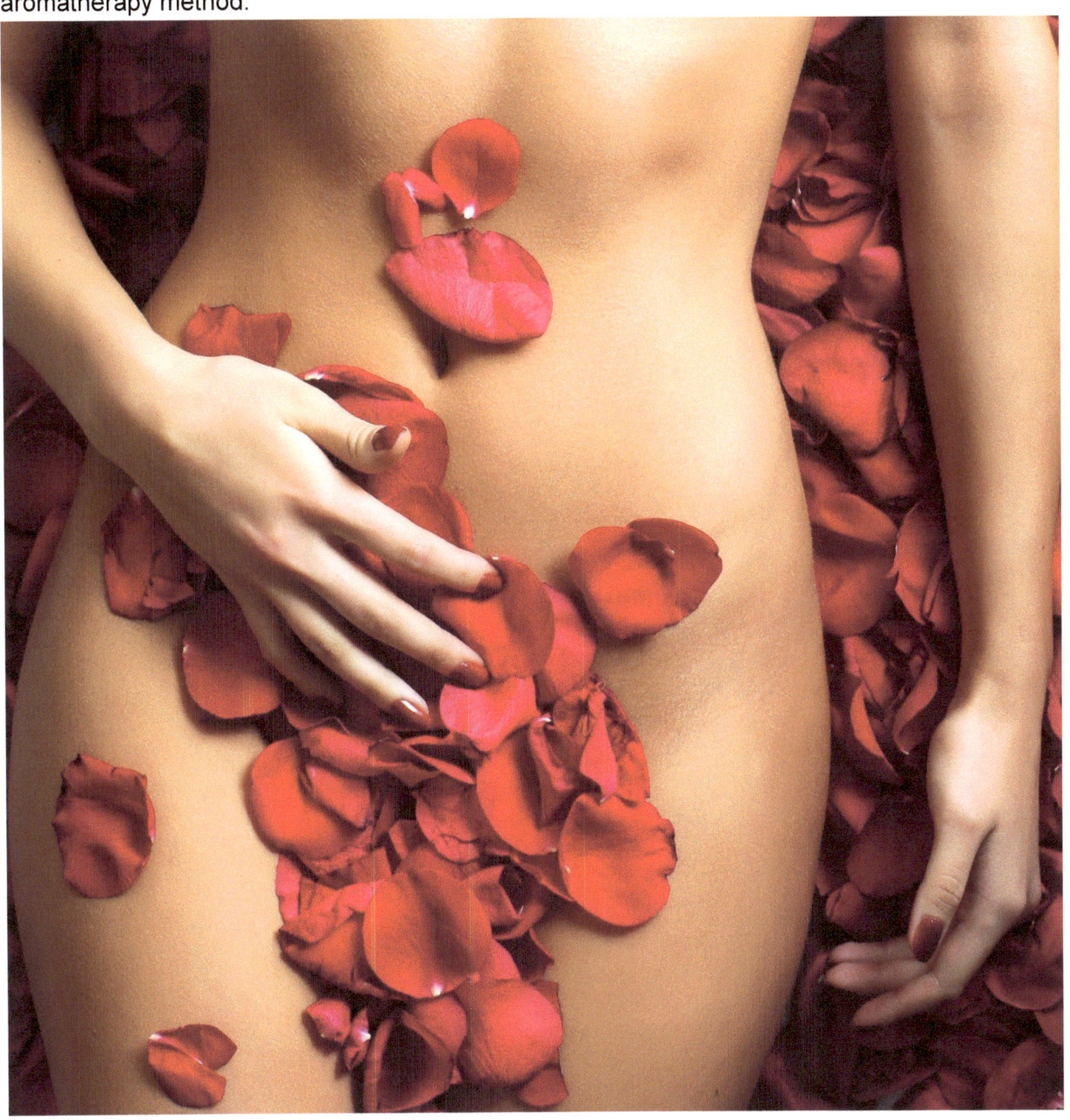

Lovers Bath oil

5 drops Sandalwood
5 drops Ylang Ylang

Mix in a 30ml bottle of almond oil and add a few drops to a bath.

Romantic Romp

6 drops Rose absolute
5 drops Jasmine
Bunch of red roses

Add the essential oils to a nice hot bath. Use with our bubble bath(following). Separate the petals and sprinkle on top of bubbles.

Lovely Bubble bath

6 drops Jasmine
6 drops ylang ylang
3 drops Rose
3 drops vanilla

4oz liquid glycrin
4 oz of castille soap
quart of water

Mix together the glycerin, water and castille soap, then add the essential oils and voila! A sexy bubble bath.

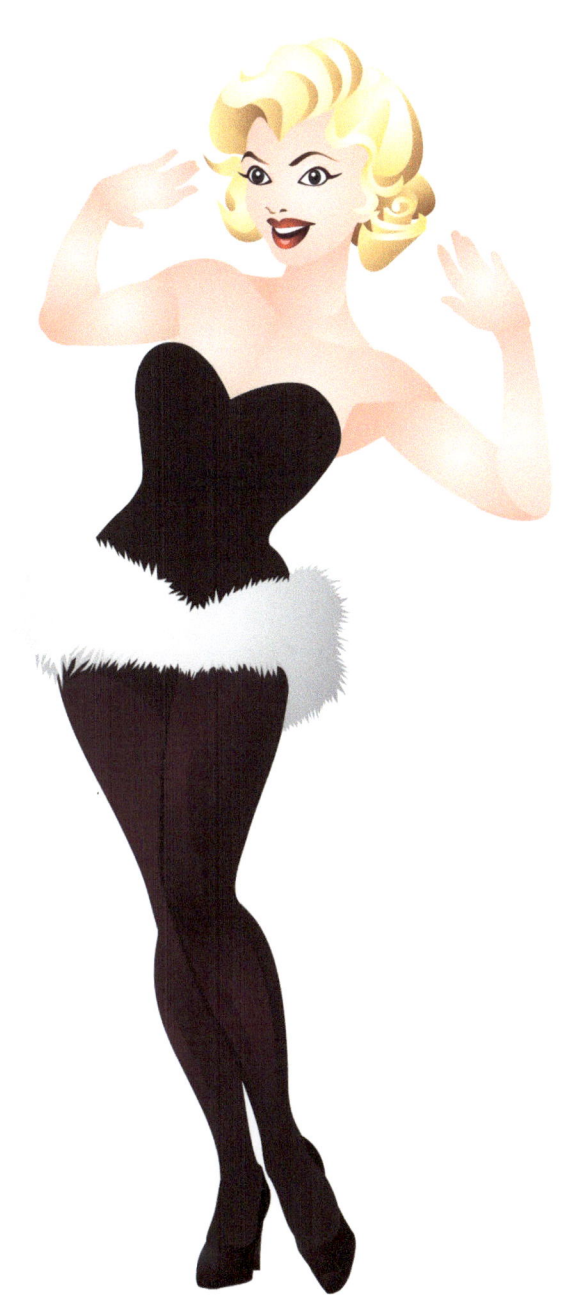

Movie Star Glam

(Uses some of the ingredients of Marylin Monroe's' favourite: Chanel no.5)

Ingeredients

4 drops rose,
4 drops jasmine,
4 drops ylang-ylang,
2 drops orange blossom,
3 drops Dutch jonquil,
2 drops Florentine iris,
4 drops tonka bean,
4 drops musk,
4 drops ginger,
4 drops amber

Method
Add the oils to 20 ml/ 70 oz perfumers alcohol or jojoba oil. You can experiment with the notes of this one with different amounts of each aroma according to your preferences.

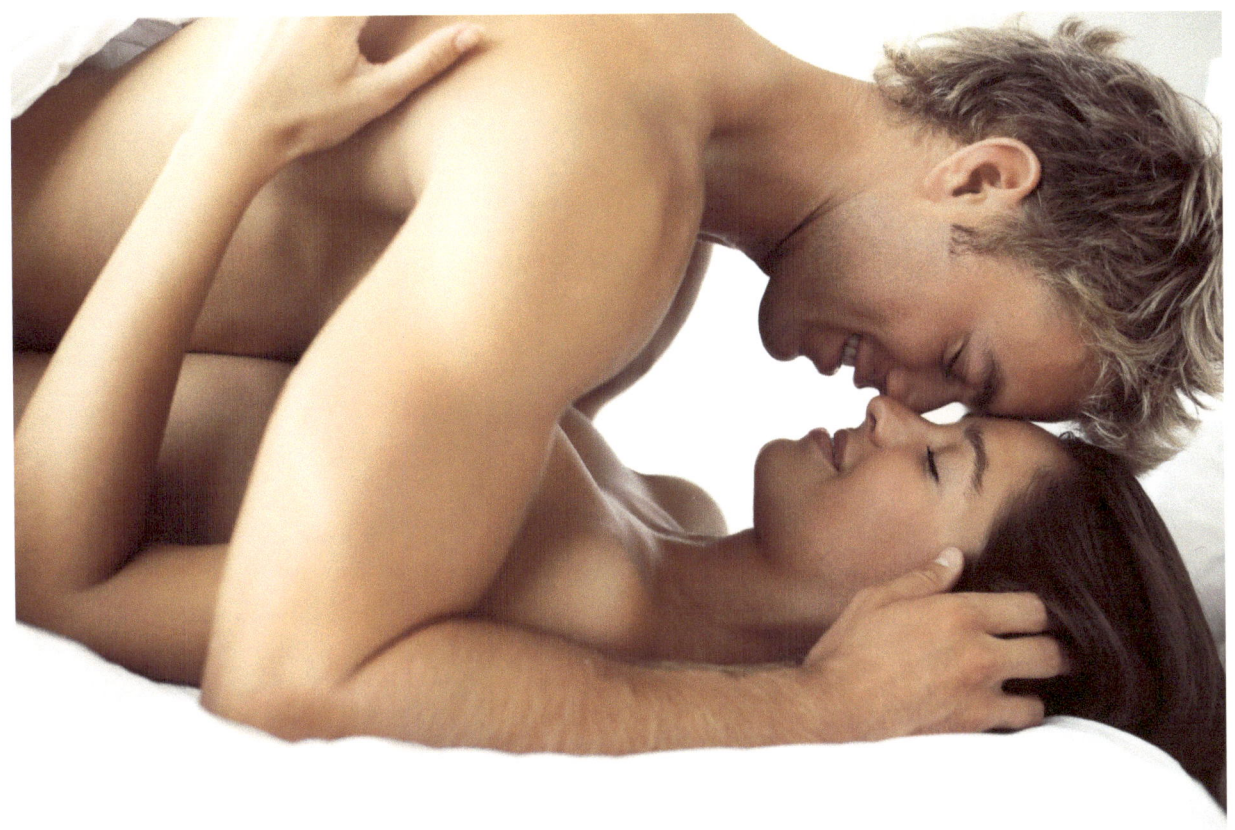

Photo: Couple in bed, Yuri Arcurs, photxpress.com

Bedroom Essentials

Ylang Ylang

Use as an anti-depressant. To treat frigidity and impotence and for balancing hormones.

Rose

For harmony, sex, and emotional problems. (Works best on women).

Jasmine

An aphrodisiac. Calms and soothes, works on impotence, frigidity and premature ejaculation.

Use these three singly or try blends using just a few drops of each in 30ml/ 1 oz of jojoba or almond oil. Or in water in an oil burner.

Eros

(A solid perfume[14])

Ingredients

1 tablespoon beeswax (available at most craft shops) or petroleum jelly
1 tablespoon Almond or Jojoba oil.
4 drops Rose
4 drops Jasmine

Method

Place the oil and the wax in a glass jar or a Pyrex bowl the place the bowl in a saucepan of water and bring to the boil. Add the essential oil to the liquid wax and stir with a fine skewer. Poor into a container with a lid. And voila! In 30 minutes it will be hardened and ready for use. If you want to make a nice perfume for a male, try this recipe replacing the rose and jasmine with some ylang ylang.

Scented Beeswax Candles.

Beeswax Sheets
Wick
20 drops (in total) of your favourite oils.

Place the wick along one edge on the beeswax sheet with the wick coming out at both ends. Carefully roll up. When you have finished gently press the edge into the candle. While you are still on the inside of the candle (near the beginning) drops some essential oils onto the wax. When rolled up trim the wick, and there you are, a lovely scented candle to romance with!

---

[14]http://www.wikihow.com/Make-Solid-Perfume (Accessed 3/07/11)

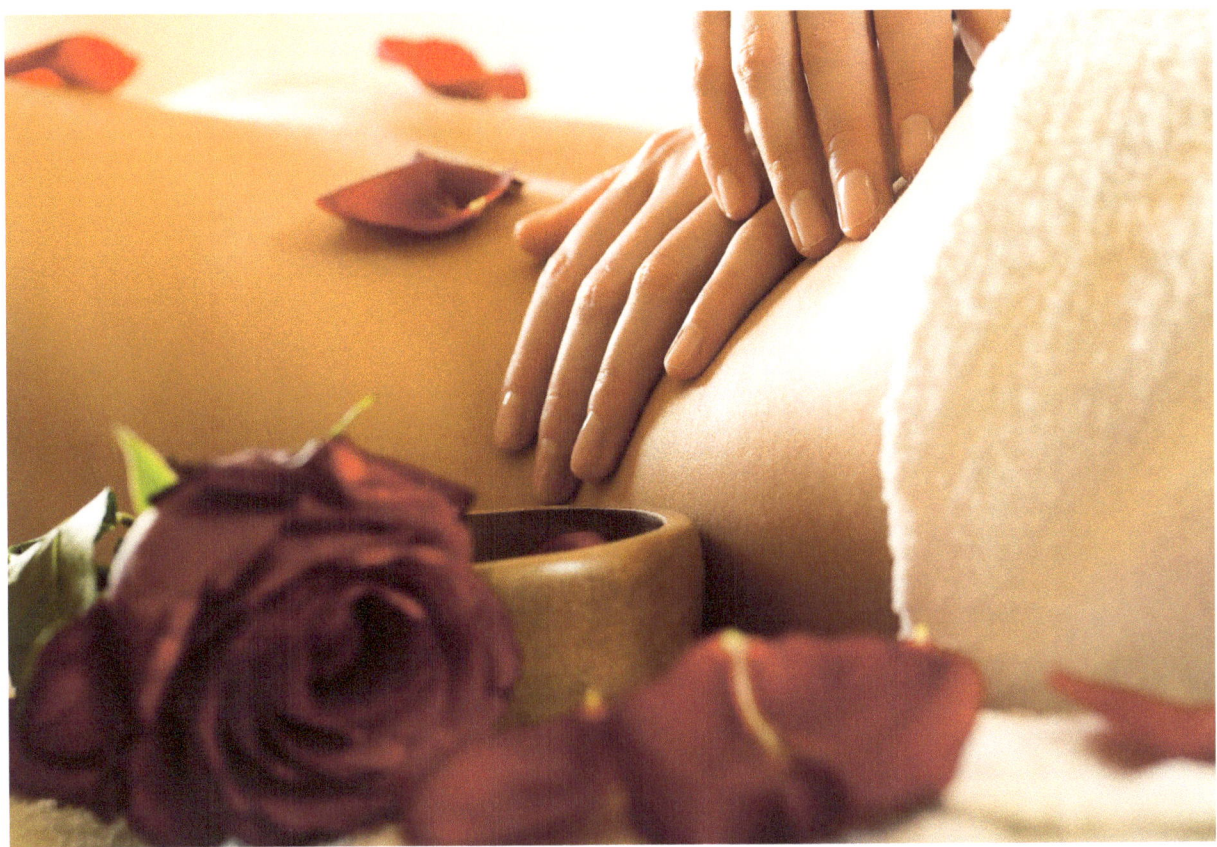

Photo: Massage, Kzenon, photoxpress.com

Scentsational Massage oil[15]

Ingredients

- One handful of Damiana leaves
- One handful of Passionflower leaves
- 8 drops Jasmine drops Ylang ylang
- 250ml/ pint Grapeseed oil

Method

Mix the herbs with the oil and bake for 3 hours. When done, strain in through some cheesecloth. Set to cool. Place in a decanter and add the ylang ylang and Jasmine oil and shake well. Voila, a sexy massage oil.You can add other scents if you wish.

---

[15]http://www.ehow.com/how_2276322_make-aphrodisiac-massage-oil.html (accessed 5/6/11)

Contraindications of Massage Therapy[16]

Do not Massage in these cases:

1. Fever
2. Inflammation
3. High blood pressure
4. Low Blood Pressure
5. Infectious diseases
6. Hernia
7. Osteoporosis
8. Varicose veins
9. Broken bones
10. Skin problems
11. Cancer
12. Other conditions and diseases: Diabetes, asthma, and other serious conditions each has its own precautions, and you should seek a doctor's opinion before administering massage.
13. HIV infection

---

[16]http://www.dummies.com/how-to/content/knowing-when-not-to-massage.html (Accessed 3/07/11)

How to Give a Sensual Massage.

Make sure your essential oils are diluted really well in a base oil. A massage table is the best way to give a massage, but otherwise your partner may lie on the floor on some blankets and you can kneel beside them. Keep them warm with towels placed over their body. Perhaps use a heater. Use one of the massage blends outlined in this book or make or buy your own. Both of you can get nude or down to your underwear, provided there is an understanding between you both that this is an erotic massage.

Start with your partner lying on their stomach. Add some oil to your hands and rub them together. Gently efflourage (long sweeping strokes) their back. Palpate (feel) for any knotty parts and try to pay more attention to these spots. Remember you can't get aroused if you're not relaxed. Use slow motion to do the massage. The best massages are done slowly. Give their trapezius and other shoulder and neck muscles a good massage. Use your thumbs, although make sure you support your own thumbs with your other hand to avoid injury, to get any knots in their shoulders out. If you feel a spot with a lot of tension you can just rest your thumb or elbow there and sink in until it releases.

Don't be to overly eager to get to the erotic parts of the massage. Although sensual massage uses gentler sweeping strokes than a remedial massage it is important to relax your subject first. All the same be gentle and romantic during the massage. You may want to play some love songs or something relaxing in the background.

After spending about 20-30 minutes on their back, cover their back with a towel and work on their legs. Don't forget their glutes. (Behind) If you notice your subject is beginning to relax now you can start to get a bit more sensuous. Men particularly like getting their glutes massaged. You can use your fists and forearms to do these big groups of muscles. After a long hard day at the office their backside really appreciates it too. While you are massaging their legs don't forget to stroke the feet.

After about ½ hour on their stomach get them to roll over onto their back. For both men and women massage the chest, they should be beginning to feel really aroused now. You can concentrate on a woman's breasts until you drive her crazy. I know most women love getting their breasts touched but not many men don't do it for long enough. So pay attention here. You can also touch the face here, which is a really intimate touch to show you love someone. Gently sweep the cheeks, and smooth the forehead. Pinch around the jawline and along the tips of the ears.

If things are really hotting up you can do body slides up and down the persons front. Support yourself on the edge of the massage table or the floor and shimmy your chest up and down their front. This is a really exciting fun part of the massage.

Once you efflourage the legs you can start massaging the more intimate parts of the body. Your lover will really like this special treat of a sensual massage. Combined with the romantic scents it will feel sensational. And you will enjoy giving the massage too.

The Essential Oils used in this Book

Amber
Bergamot
Blood Orange
Blue Lotus
Cinnamon
Clary Sage
Ginger
Grapefruit
Jasmine
Jonquil
Iris
Lemon
Musk
Mandarin
Myrtle
Neroli
Orange blossom
Patchouli
Rose Absolute
Rose Otto
Rosewood
Sandalwood
Tangarine
Tonka bean
Vanilla
Violet
Ylang Ylang

The Oils and their Properties for Use with this Book.

The notes in essential oils, comparable to the musical scale, were classified by a Frenchman called Piesse in the 19th C.

The formula usually used is to use less of the top notes and more of the middle notes and even more of the base notes.

A round fragrance would usually use the following percentages:

20% top note
30% middle note
50% base note.

Of course the fragrance must be diluted in a carrier oil, perfumers alcohol or water. You only need about a half or quarter the amount of essential drops to the carrier oil. As we age the dilution is stronger[17]. The rules can always be broken to suit your temperament or needs.

Here is a basic perfume recipe sourced from About.com. So you can play with the notes as outlined on the following pages.

How to Make Perfume

"15 ml/ 1/2 ounce Jojoba oil or sweet almond oil
75 ml/ 2-1/2 ounces ethanol (e.g., vodka)
2 tablespoons spring water or distilled water (not tap water)
coffee filter
dark-colored glass bottle
25 drops essential oils (buy them at a health store or online or distill your own)
 7 drops base note essential oils
 7 drops middle note essential oils
 6-7 drops top note essential oils
 couple of drops of bridge notes (optional)

1. *Add the jojoba oil or sweet almond oil to the bottle.*
2. *Add the essential oils in the following order: the base notes, followed by the middle notes, then finally the top notes. Add a couple of drops of bridge notes, if desired".*
3. *Add 2-1/2 ounces of alcohol.*

---

[17]http://www.essentialoils.co.za/blending_fragrances.htm (Accessed 1/07/11)

4. *Shake the bottle for a couple of minutes then let it sit for 48 hours to 6 weeks. The scent will change over time, becoming strongest around 6 weeks.*

5. *When the scent is where you want it to be, add 2 tablespoons of spring water to the perfume. Shake the bottle to mix the perfume, then filter it through a coffee filter and pour it into its final bottle. Ideally, this will be a dark bottle with minimal airspace, since light and exposure to air degrade many essential oils.*

6. *You can pour a little perfume into a decorative bottle, but in general, store your perfume in a dark sealed bottle, away from heat and light.*

7. *Label your creation. It's a good idea to record how you made the perfume, in case you want to duplicate it"*[18].

---

[18] http://chemistry.about.com/od/chemistryhowtoguide/a/makeperfume.htm (Accessed 1/07/11)

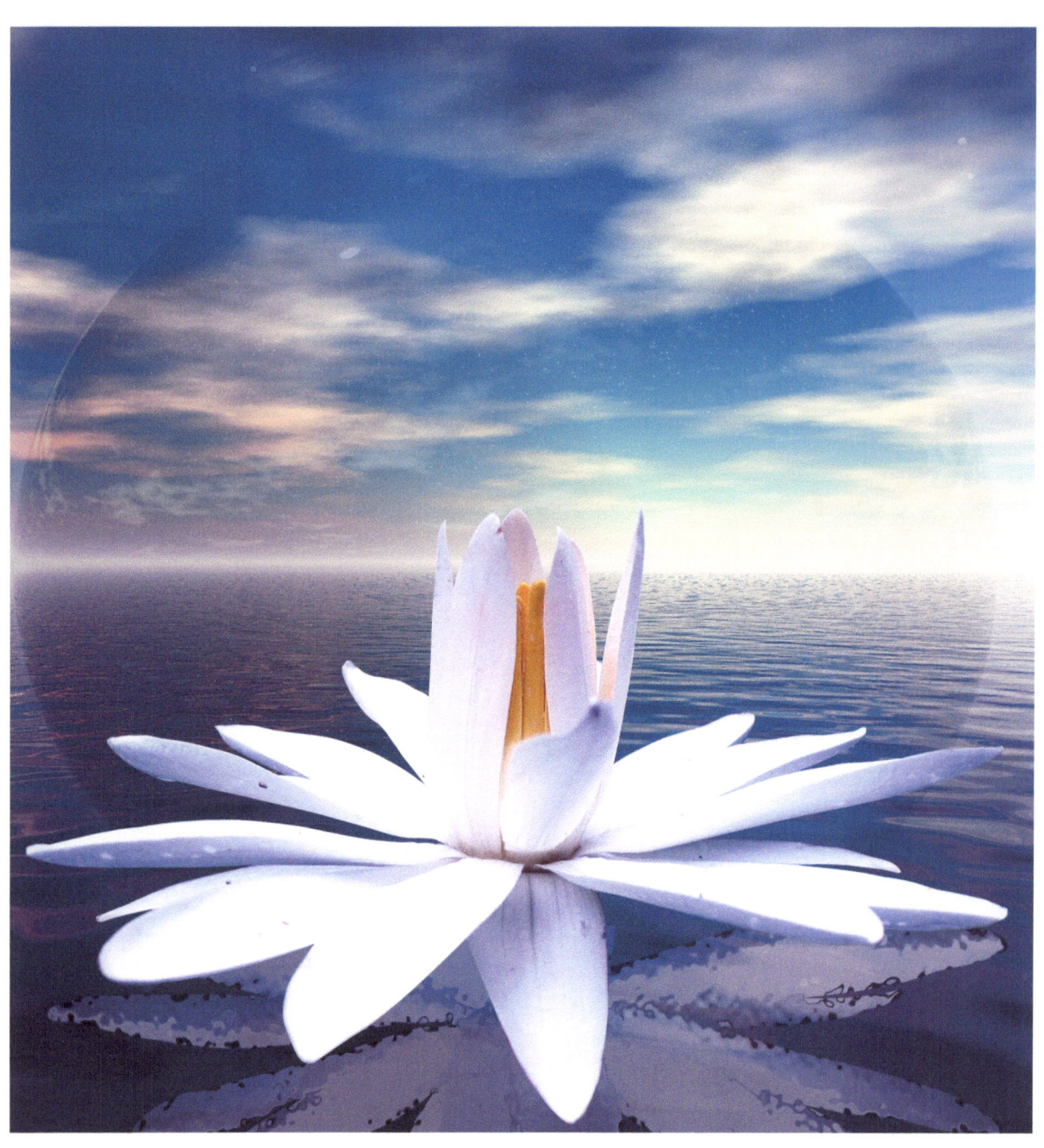

Photo: Lotus, RGB Space, photoxpress.com

Amber Calming.	Base note.
Bergamot Happiness	Top note.
Blood Orange Anti-depressant, aphrodisiac, uplifting and stimulating.	Top note.
Blue Lotus Intoxicating, sexual enhancer.	Middle note.
Cedarwood Aphrodisiac.	Base note.
Cinnamon Invigorating, rejuvenating.	Top note.
Clary Sage Relaxing and sedating.	Top note.
Frankincense Soothing	Base note
Ginger Gentle, stimulating.	Base note.

Grapefruit Refreshing, uplifting.	Top note.
Iris Sedative.	Top note.
Jasmine Uplifting and stimulating .	Base note.
Jonquil Used in perfumery, Insipration.	Middle note.
Lavender Calming, relaxing and balancing.	Middle note.
Lemon Refreshing	Top note.
Musk Power, aphrodisiac.	Base note.
Mandarin Happiness, joy, aphrodisiac.	Top note.

Myrtle Soothing	Middle note.
Neroli Lift spirits and clear the mind.	Top note.
Orange blossom Love.	Top note.
Patchouli Tonic and stimulant.	Base note.
Rose Absolute Balance and harmony	Base note.
Rose Otto See Rose.	Base note.
Rosewood Good for skin	Base note.
Tangarine	Top note.

Eases tension	
Sandalwood Aphrodisiac	Base note
Tonka bean Aphrodisiac, euphoric	Base note.
Vanilla Passion.	Base note.
Vetiver Helps with stress.	Base note.
Violet Passion.	Top note.
Ylang Ylang Calming balancing and relaxing.	Base note

For Aromatherapy Suppliers or to find out more about the author, visit my website
www.maree-celestebonnet.tk

Bibliography

http://www.mnwelldir.org/docs/therapies/essentia02.htm (Accessed 1/07/11)

http://www.essential7.com/essential_oil_profiles/profiles/amber_oil.html (accessed 1/07/11)

http://www.newdirectionsaromatics.com/blood-orange-essential-oil-p-189.html (Accessed 1/07/11)

http://www.shamansgarden.com/c-13-blue-lilylotus.aspx (Accessed 1/07/11)

http://en.wikipedia.org/wiki/Iris_%28plant%29 (Accessed 1/07/11)

http://www.gritman.com/tonka-bean-essential-oil.html (Accessed 1/07/11)

http://www.aromatherapygoddess.com/essentialoilproperties.html (Accessed 1/07/11)

http://www.essentialoils.co.za/blending_fragrances.htm (Accessed 1/07/11)

http://www.gardenguides.com/86361-information-jonquil-flowers.html (Accessed 1/07/11)

https://www.dshperfumes.com/ozone_eo.asp?page=6 (Accessed 1/07/11)

http://www.beauty-tips.net/aromaticstips/essentialoils/essential-oils-top-middle-base-notes.htm#axzz1QpvfiwZC

http://www.aromaweb.com/essential-oils/atlas-cedarwood-oil.asp (Accessed 3/07/11)

The End